SPOTLIGHT ON OUR FUTURE

PHYSICAL HEALTH
IN OUR WORLD

JANARI AUDRA

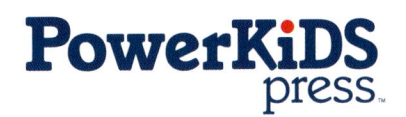

NEW YORK

Published in 2022 by The Rosen Publishing Group, Inc.
29 East 21st Street, New York, NY 10010

First Edition

Editor: Theresa Emminizer
Book Design: Michael Flynn

Photo Credits: Cover LightField Studios/Shutterstock.com; (series background) jessicahyde/Shutterstock.com; p. 4 FatCamera/E+/Getty Images; p. 5 Jose Luis Pelaez Inc/DigitalVision/Getty Images; p. 7 DEA/A.DAGLI ORTI/De Agostini/Getty Images; p. 8 Fine Art/Corbis Historical/Getty Images; p. 9 Print Collector/Hulton Archive/Getty Images; p. 11 Popperfoto/Getty Images; p. 12 Maxx-Studio/Shutterstock.com; p. 13 Mohammed Hammoud/Getty Images; pp. 14, 15 Adam Jan Figel/Shutterstock.com; p. 16 Digital Images Studio/Shutterstock.com; p. 17 MLADEN ANTONOV/AFP/Getty Images; p. 19 (cancer cell) jovan vitanovski/Shutterstock.com; p. 19 (Rishab Jain) https://en.wikipedia.org/wiki/Rishab_Jain#/media/File:RishabJain_2018.jpg; p. 20 Hung Chung Chih/Shutterstock.com; p. 21 STR/Stringer/AFP/Getty Images; p. 22 Anna Om/Shutterstock.com; p. 23 ISSOUF SANOGO/AFP/Getty Images; p. 25 hadynyah/E+/Getty Images; p. 26 Valeri Potapova/Shutterstock.com; p. 27 OLYMPIA DE MAISMONT/AFP/Getty Images; p. 28 Andrey_Popov/Shutterstock.com; p. 29 RUTH MCDOWALL/AFP/Getty Images.

Some of the images in this book illustrate individuals who are models. The depictions do not imply actual situations or events.

Cataloging-in-Publication Data

Names: Audra, Janari.
Title: Physical health in our world / Janari Audra.
Description: New York : PowerKids Press, 2022. | Series: Spotlight on our future | Includes glossary and index.
Identifiers: ISBN 9781725324152 (pbk.) | ISBN 9781725324183 (library bound) | ISBN 9781725324169 (6 pack)
Subjects: LCSH: Health--Juvenile literature. | Health attitudes--Juvenile literature. | Medicine, Preventive--Juvenile literature. | Vaccination--Juvenile literature.
Classification: LCC RA777.A93 2022 | DDC 613--dc23

Manufactured in the United States of America

CPSIA Compliance Information: Batch #CSPK22. For further information contact Rosen Publishing, New York, New York at 1-800-237-9932.

Find us on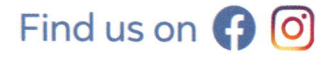

CONTENTS

CHAPTER ONE

GOALS FOR BETTER HEALTH

Did you know that over 95 percent of the world's population suffers from at least one health problem? Many illnesses can be cured, but some can't. Physical, or bodily, health is an important issue around the world. Not enough people have the care they need to stay healthy. They may be living where there's poor health care or few doctors. Even where there are many doctors, some people may not be educated about health.

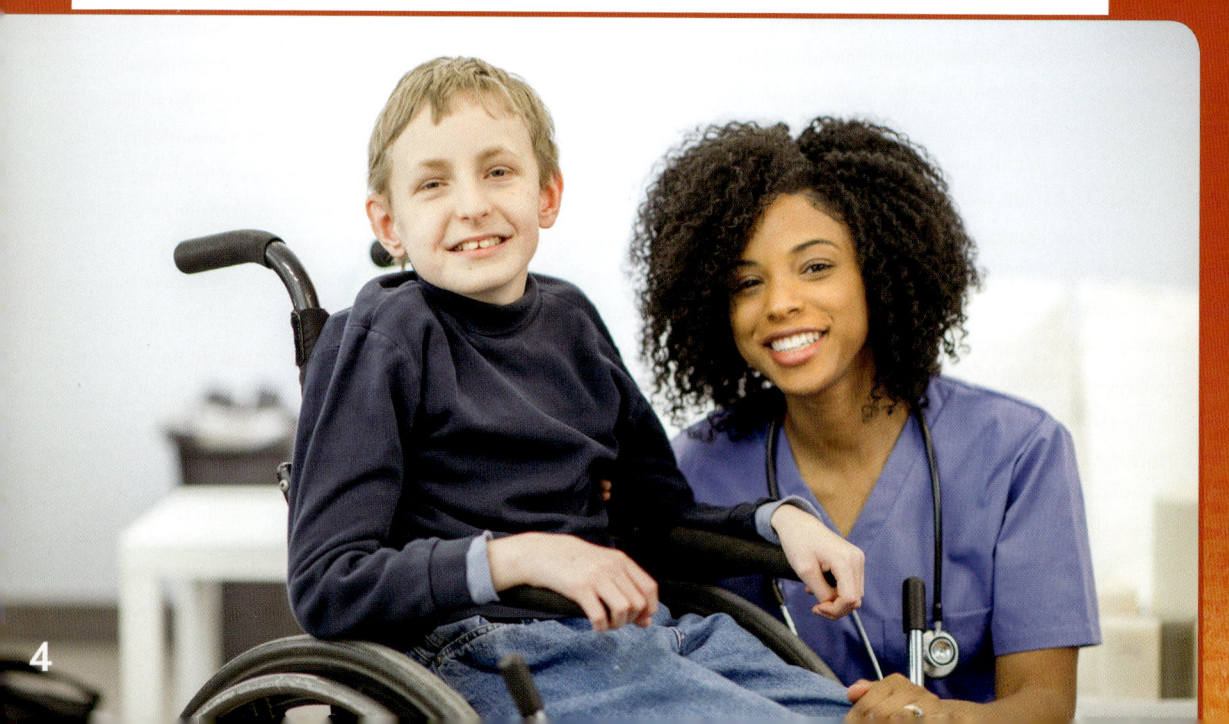

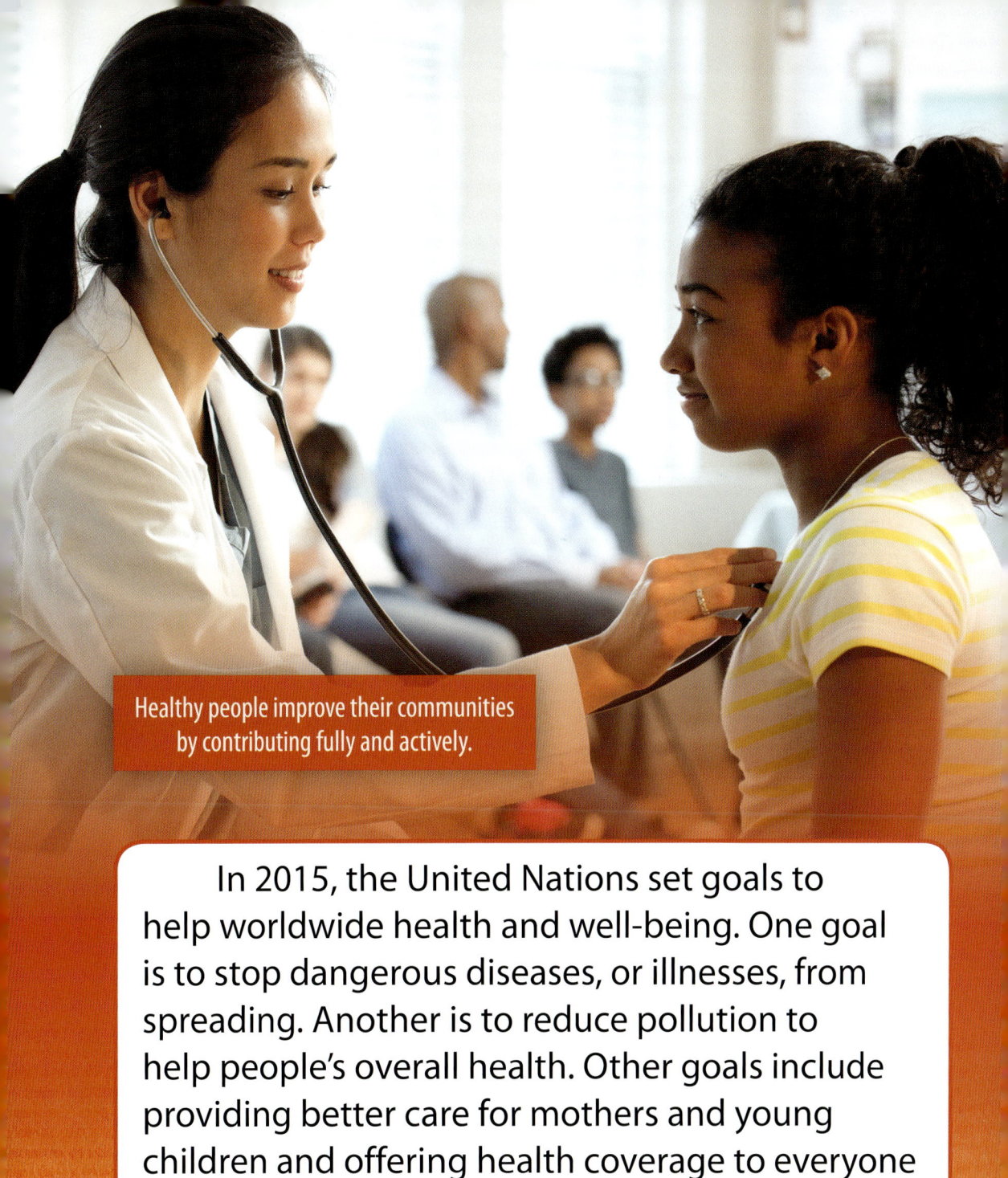

Healthy people improve their communities by contributing fully and actively.

In 2015, the United Nations set goals to help worldwide health and well-being. One goal is to stop dangerous diseases, or illnesses, from spreading. Another is to reduce pollution to help people's overall health. Other goals include providing better care for mothers and young children and offering health coverage to everyone throughout the world.

CHAPTER TWO

A HISTORY OF DISEASE

Disease and illness have always been part of human life. Sometimes illnesses spread between humans and animals. Other times, people became ill because they were missing key **nutrients** in their diets. Some diseases pass very easily between people. A lack of cleanliness has also made large numbers of people ill.

In ancient Greece, a doctor named Hippocrates studied disease. He suggested that diseases happened because of imbalances in the body or because of problems in the **environment**. Hippocrates also saw a difference between what we now call epidemic diseases and endemic diseases. Epidemics are widespread diseases that spread quickly from one person to another. Endemic diseases are limited to a certain area. These terms are still used by doctors today.

Hippocrates is known as the father of medicine.

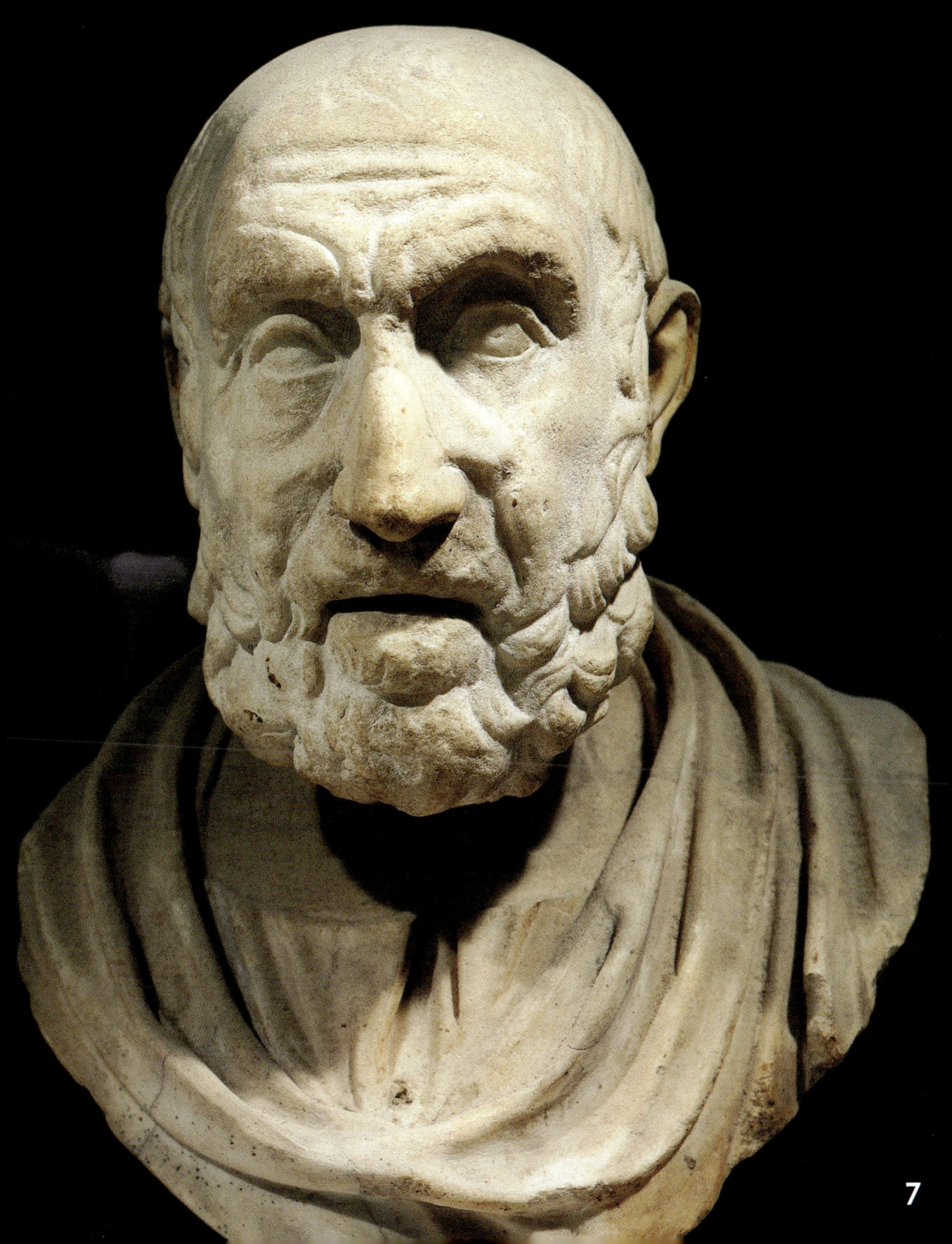

CHAPTER THREE

PUBLIC HEALTH BEGINS

Many of the diseases of the Middle Ages were caused by poor living conditions. Garbage and waste piled up in cities. This attracted rats. The rats helped spread diseases such as **plague**. Crowded living conditions also cause diseases to spread quickly from person to person.

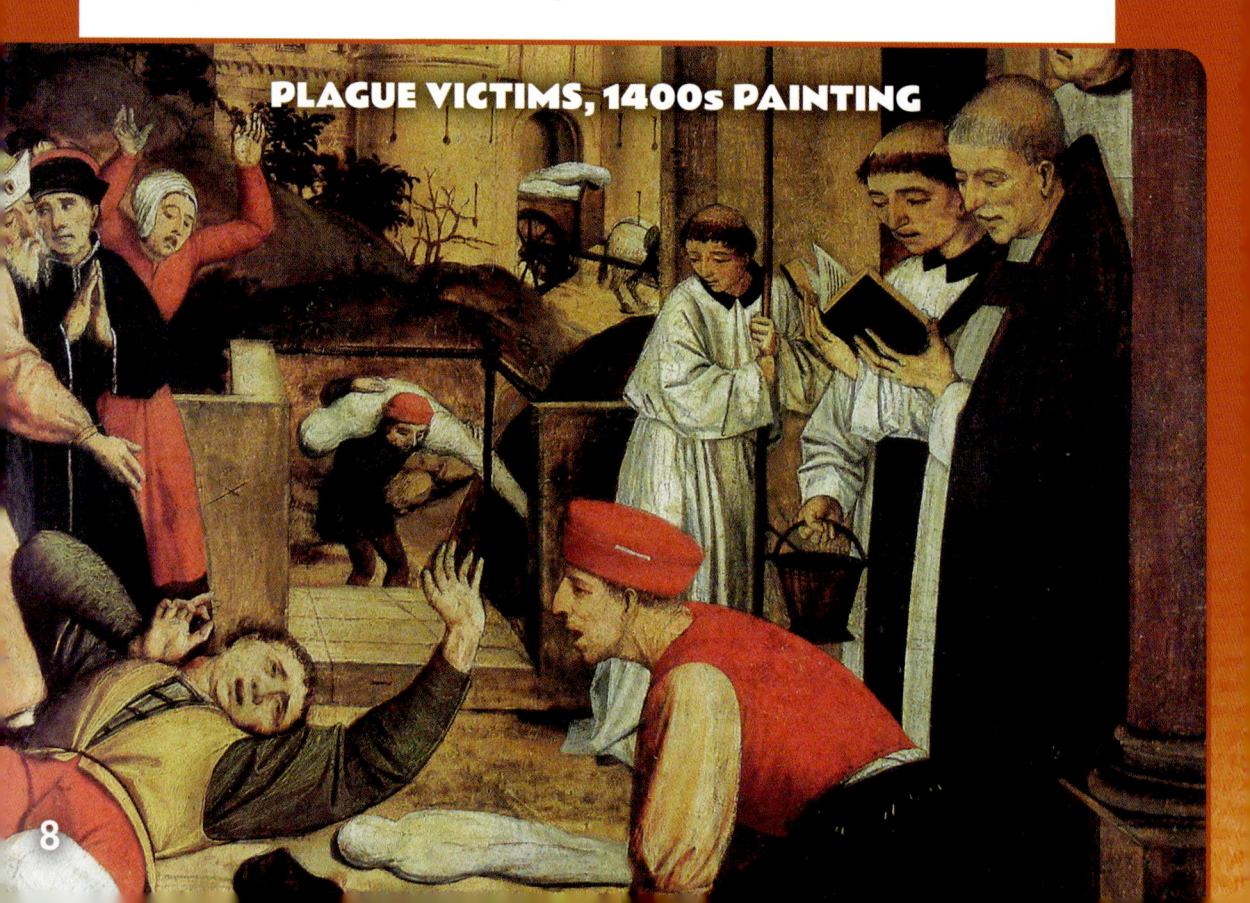

PLAGUE VICTIMS, 1400s PAINTING

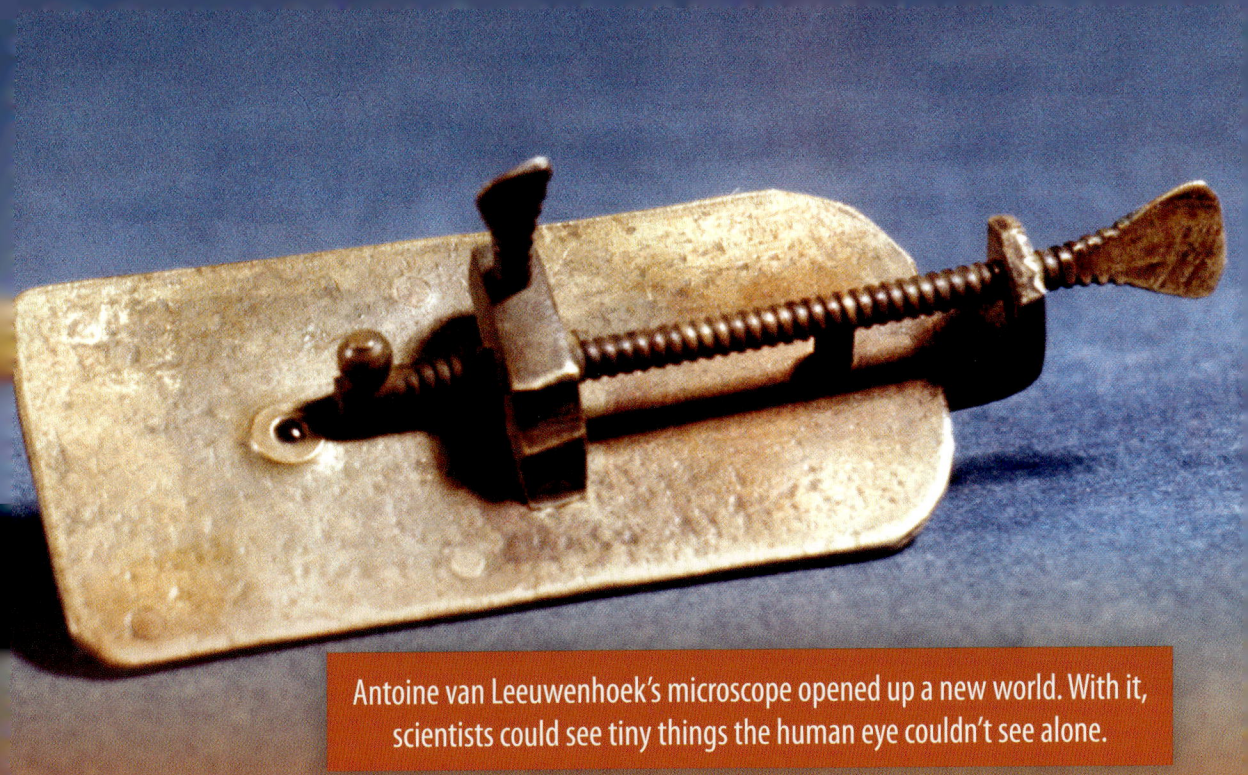

Antoine van Leeuwenhoek's microscope opened up a new world. With it, scientists could see tiny things the human eye couldn't see alone.

Technology helped people understand disease. In the 1670s, scientist Antoine van Leeuwenhoek was the first to view bacteria through a microscope. This helped scientists learn how tiny bacteria could harm the human body.

Then, in the 1700s, an important idea took hold. People began thinking that good governments helped with a society's good health. They realized that it was important to have healthy citizens. A healthy society, they thought, would also help the economy. Today, this idea is known as public health.

CHAPTER FOUR

THE FIRST HOSPITALS

In the 1700s and 1800s, hospitals opened across Europe and North America. They helped the sick, and they also became places for medical training and study.

Throughout the 20th century, people made new discoveries. Hospitals became safer, and doctors and scientists discovered newer medicines and treatments. These new advances saved many lives.

There's been amazing progress in medicine and public health, but more needs to be done. Malnutrition, or poor nutrition, is still a major problem in many places. Diseases such as AIDS and malaria kill many people around the world. Solving these problems means improving living conditions for many people. It also means improving access to health care in many areas. More research is also needed. Scientists haven't found cures for illnesses such as cancer and heart disease.

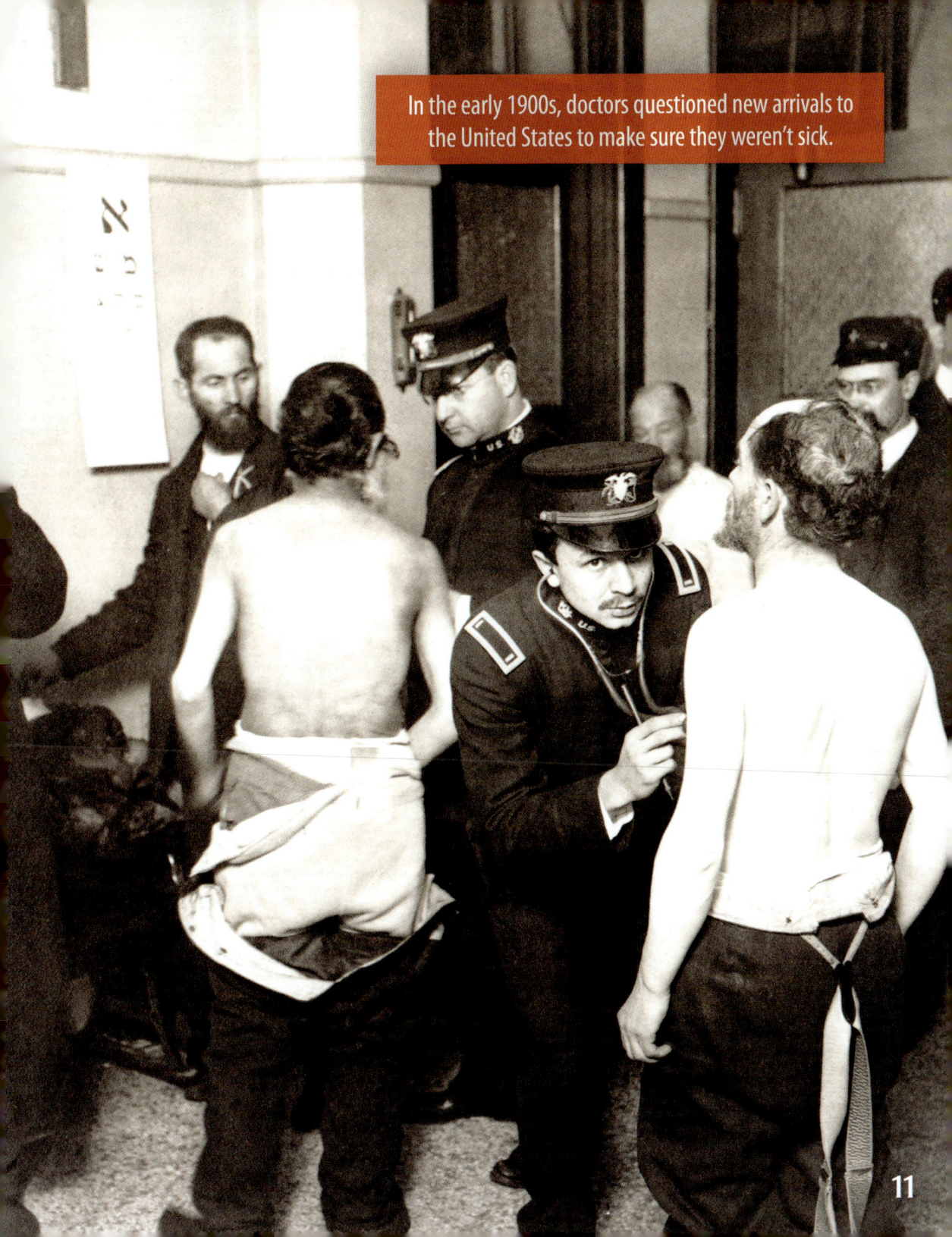

In the early 1900s, doctors questioned new arrivals to the United States to make sure they weren't sick.

CHAPTER FIVE

THE POWER OF VACCINES

Vaccines are some of the most powerful tools available for improving public health. A vaccine gives the patient limited exposure to specific germs. When the body fights off these germs, it may keep the person from getting the disease in the future.

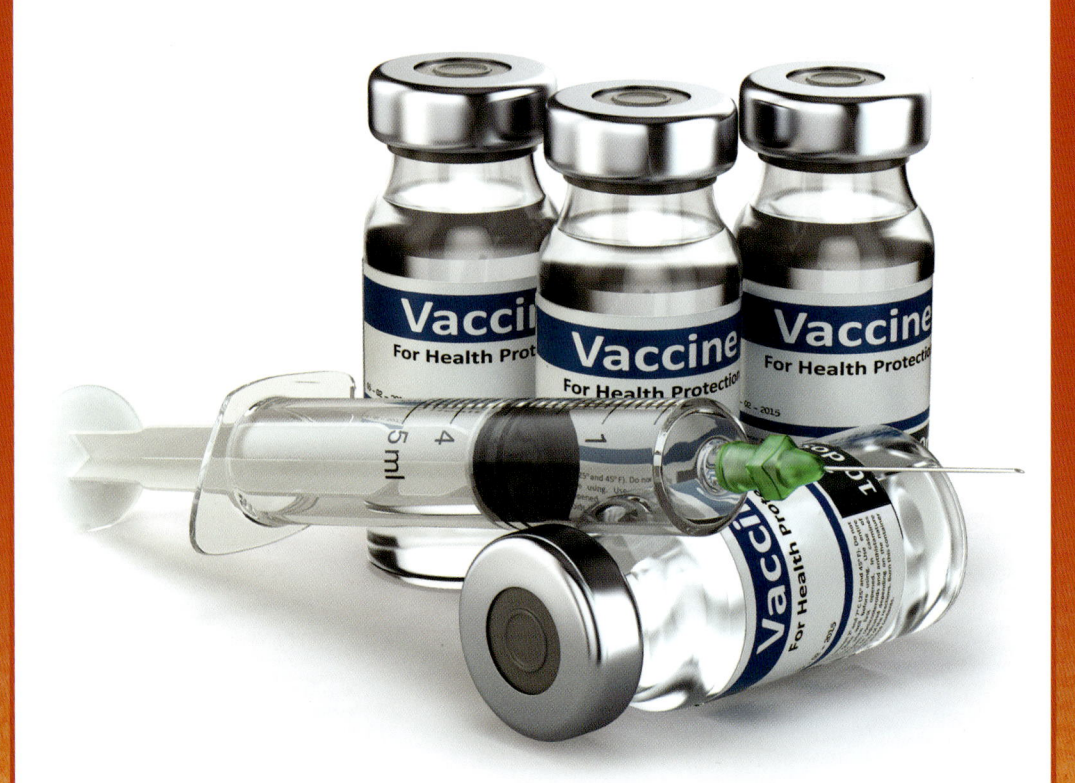

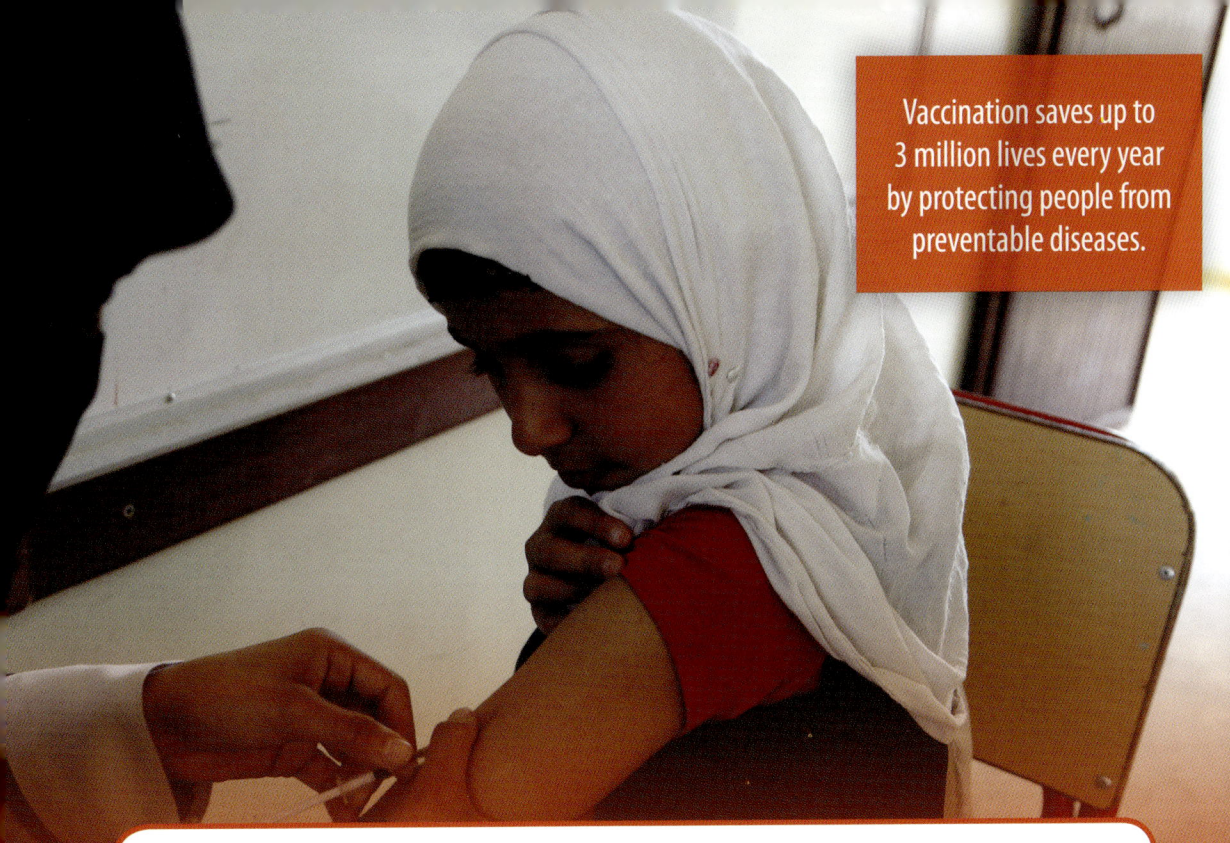

Vaccination saves up to 3 million lives every year by protecting people from preventable diseases.

British doctor Edward Jenner developed the first modern vaccine in 1796. It helped prevent a deadly disease called smallpox. As time went on, smallpox vaccinations became more available. By 1979, the disease was officially eliminated, or done away with.

In 1955, American scientist Jonas Salk perfected the vaccine for another deadly disease, polio, which often affects children. It can lead to **paralysis** or death. Salk's vaccine protected people from the disease. Today, vaccines can prevent many dangerous diseases.

CHAPTER SIX

HIV AND AIDS

One of the most serious health problems in the world today is the virus HIV, which leads to another illness called AIDS. The virus attacks the body's immune system, which helps people fight disease naturally. If left untreated, HIV leads to AIDS. This disease weakens the body even more, and many infections can lead to death. About 32 million people have died from AIDS since it was first identified in 1983.

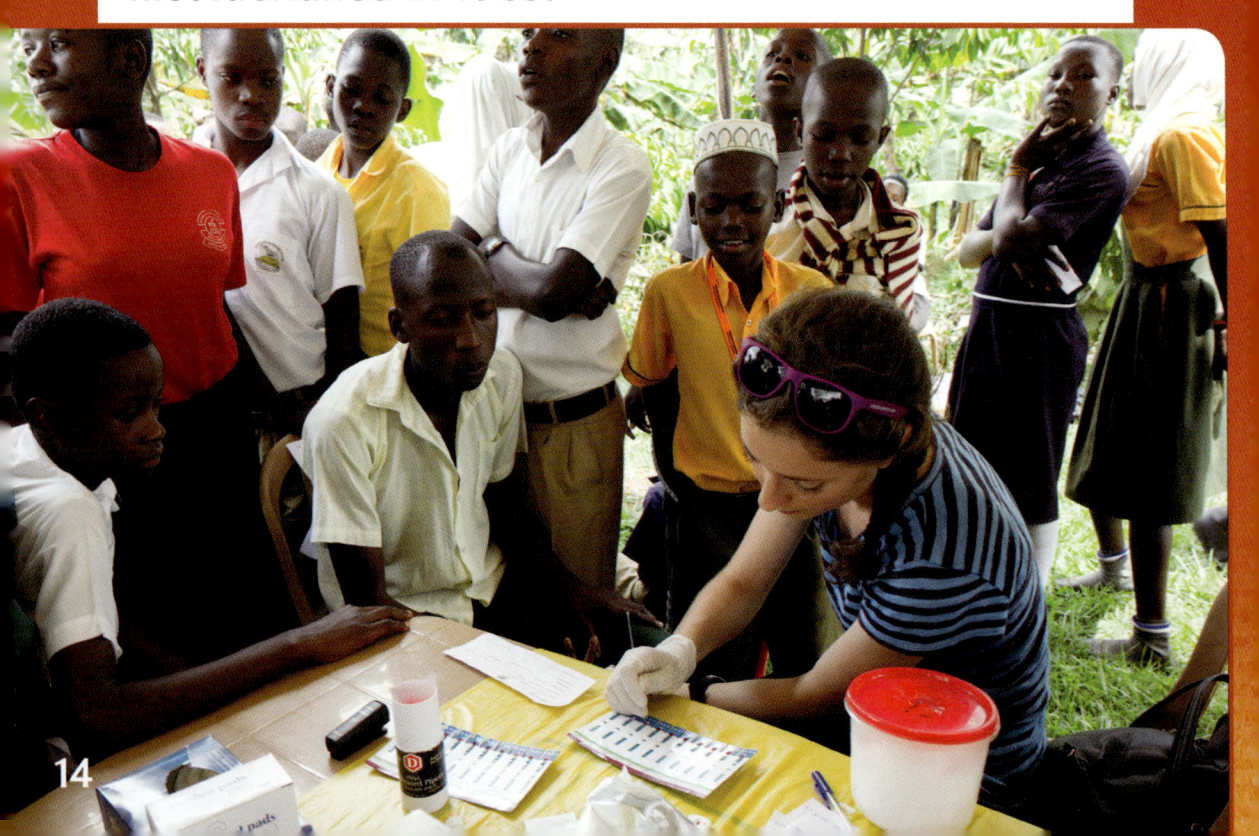

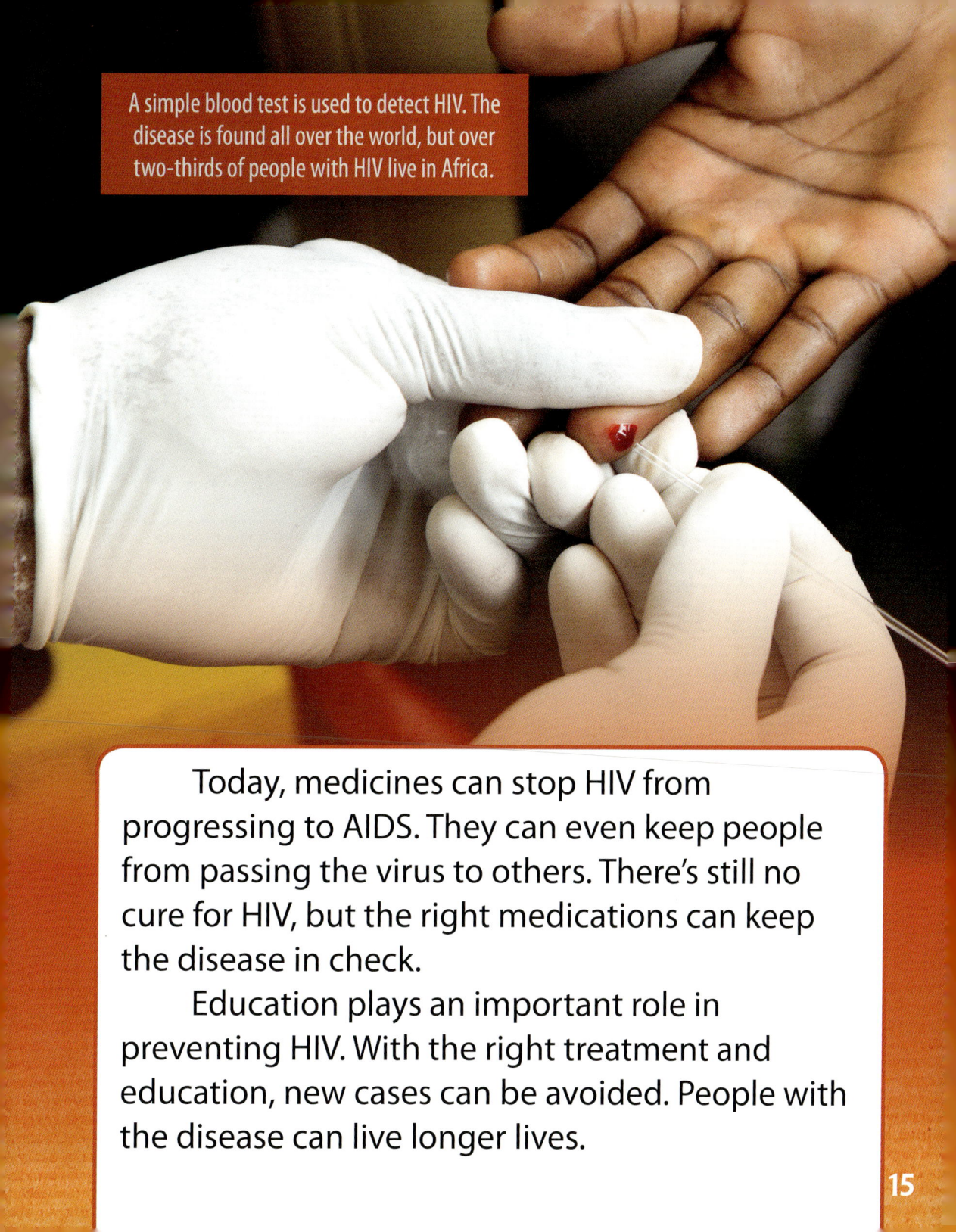

A simple blood test is used to detect HIV. The disease is found all over the world, but over two-thirds of people with HIV live in Africa.

Today, medicines can stop HIV from progressing to AIDS. They can even keep people from passing the virus to others. There's still no cure for HIV, but the right medications can keep the disease in check.

Education plays an important role in preventing HIV. With the right treatment and education, new cases can be avoided. People with the disease can live longer lives.

CHAPTER SEVEN

OTHER DISEASES

There are other deadly diseases that affect the world. Tuberculosis is a disease that's caused by bacteria that are passed through the air. About 1.5 million people died from the disease in 2018. However, vaccines and medicine can prevent and cure it.

With the deadly disease called malaria, mosquito bites pass **parasites** to people. Malaria mostly affects people in developing countries. There were 405,000 deaths from malaria in 2018. There are ways to prevent the disease, however, and doctors are trying to get rid of it worldwide.

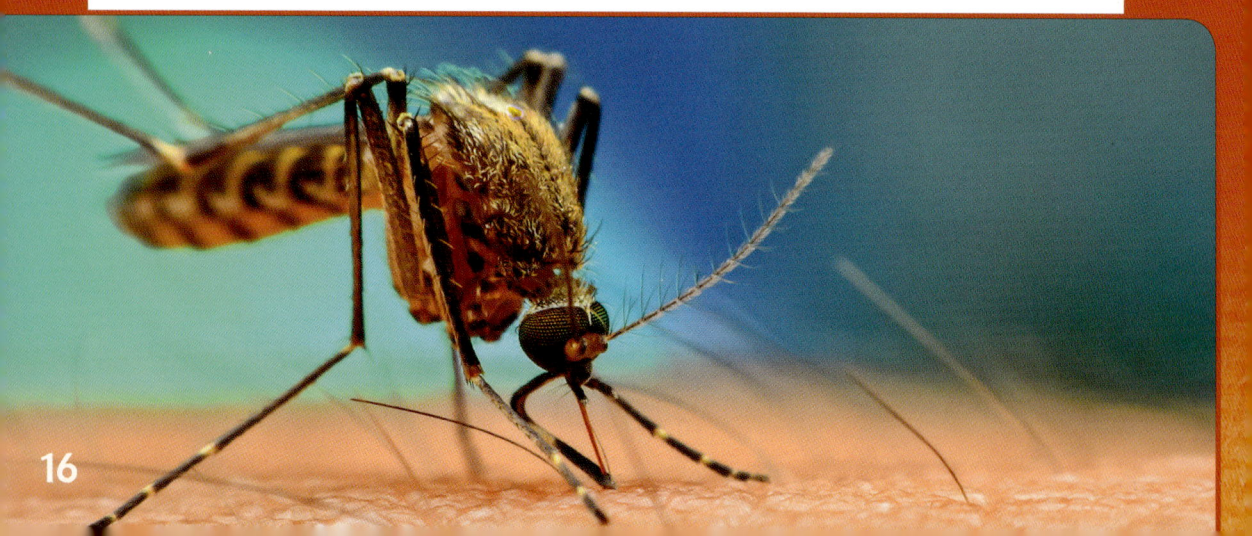

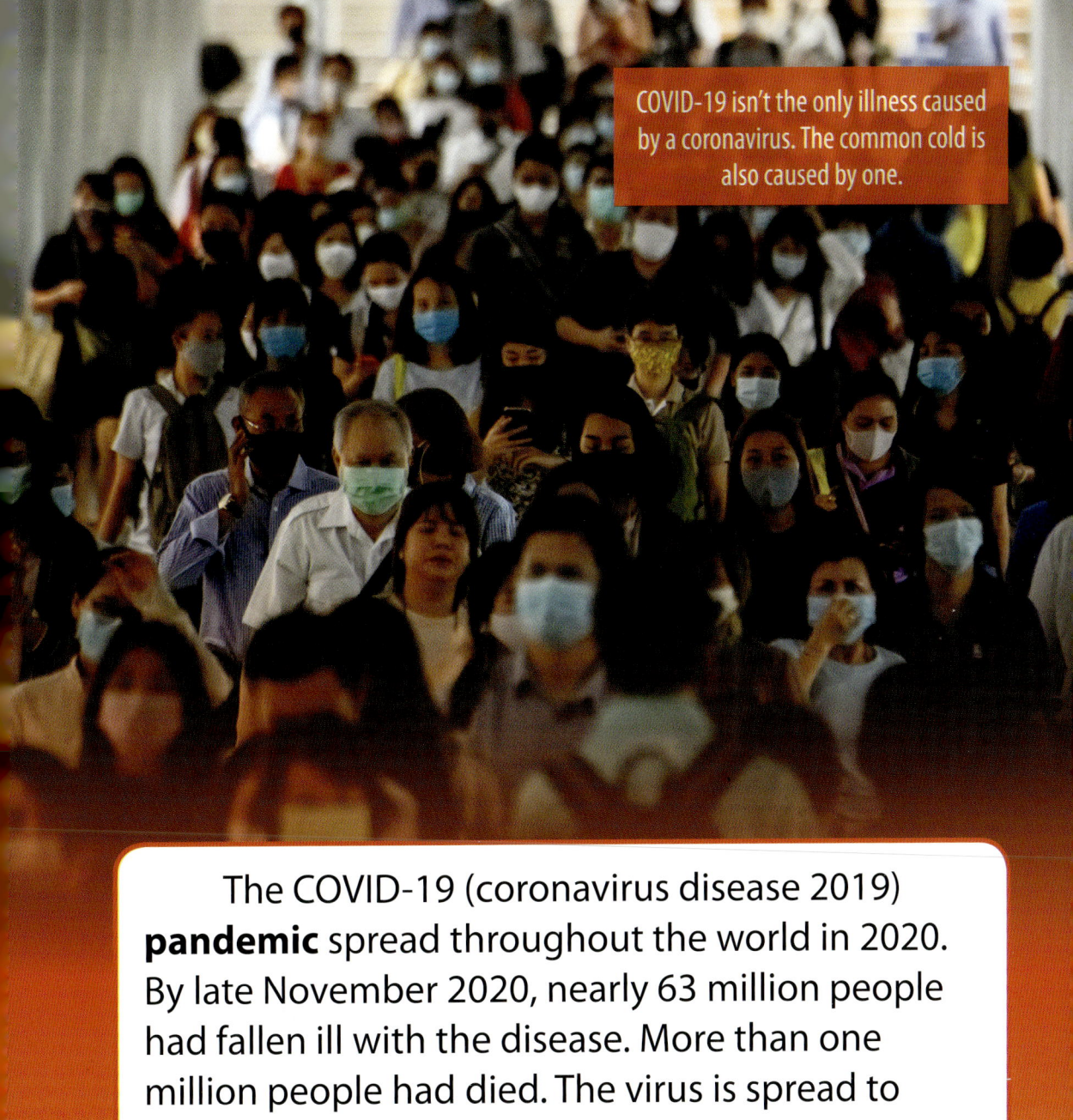

COVID-19 isn't the only illness caused by a coronavirus. The common cold is also caused by one.

The COVID-19 (coronavirus disease 2019) **pandemic** spread throughout the world in 2020. By late November 2020, nearly 63 million people had fallen ill with the disease. More than one million people had died. The virus is spread to others when people cough or sneeze. Scientists around the world urged people to wear masks and practice social distancing, but the pandemic lasted for many months.

CHAPTER EIGHT

HEART DISEASE, DIABETES, AND CANCER

Not all diseases are communicable, or able to be spread from person to person. Other diseases include heart disease, diabetes, and cancer. Sometimes people are more likely to suffer from certain diseases because of **genetics**. These diseases are often linked to poverty. Unhealthy diet and lack of exercise can lead to these illnesses.

Heart disease is the number one cause of death worldwide. Diabetes is also very common. It involves the body's ability to make **insulin**. In 2019, 463 million adults had diabetes.

Cancer is caused by abnormal, or unnatural, cell growth. It can happen in different parts of the body and is hard to treat. The earlier it's found, the better it can be treated.

When he was in eighth grade, Rishab Jain developed new technology to help treat cancer.

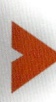

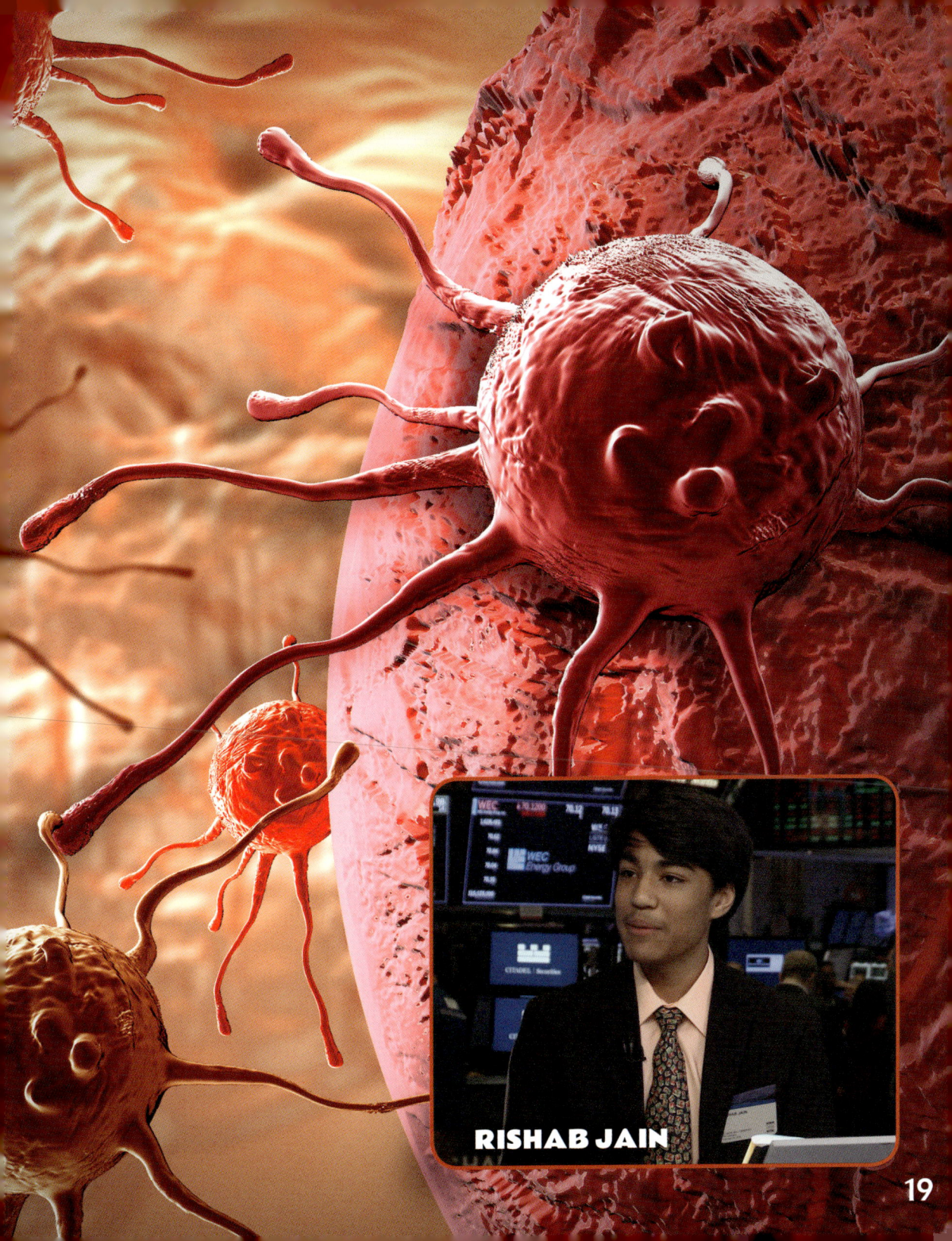

RISHAB JAIN

CHAPTER NINE

THE POLLUTION PROBLEM

Many diseases are related to environmental factors around us. For example, air pollution causes about 7 million deaths a year. It causes about 30 percent of deaths from strokes, lung cancer, or heart disease. Air pollution can also cause a condition called asthma.

Air pollution can happen in many ways. For example, factories and cars put smoke and tiny bits of pollution into the air. Some of these bits are so small they can pass from the lungs into the blood stream.

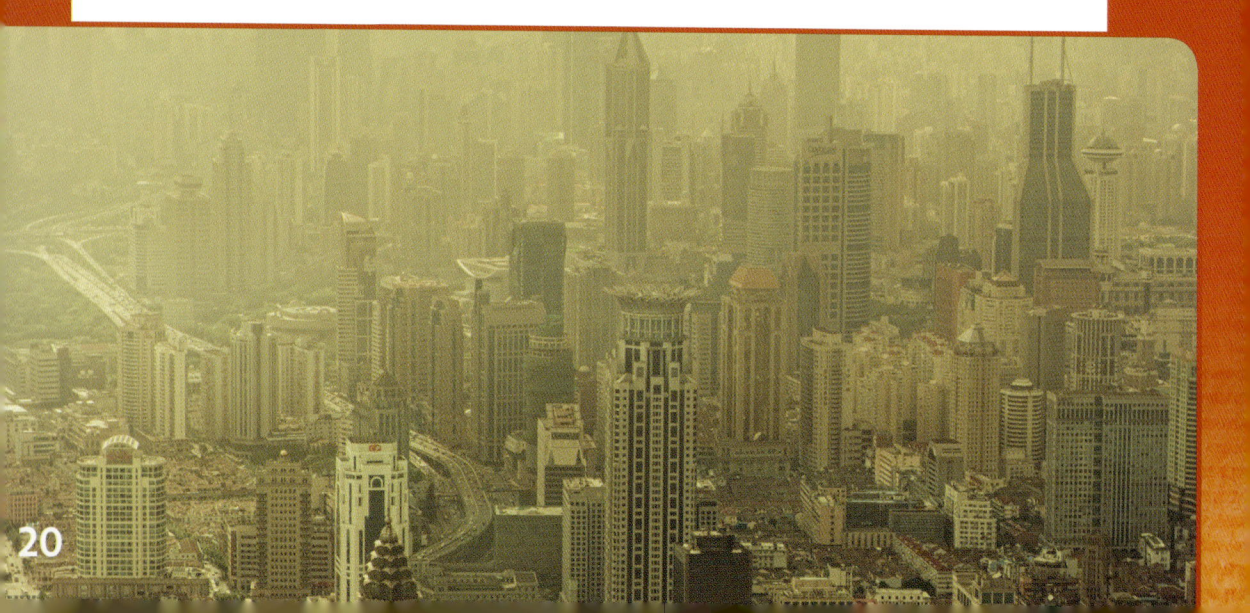

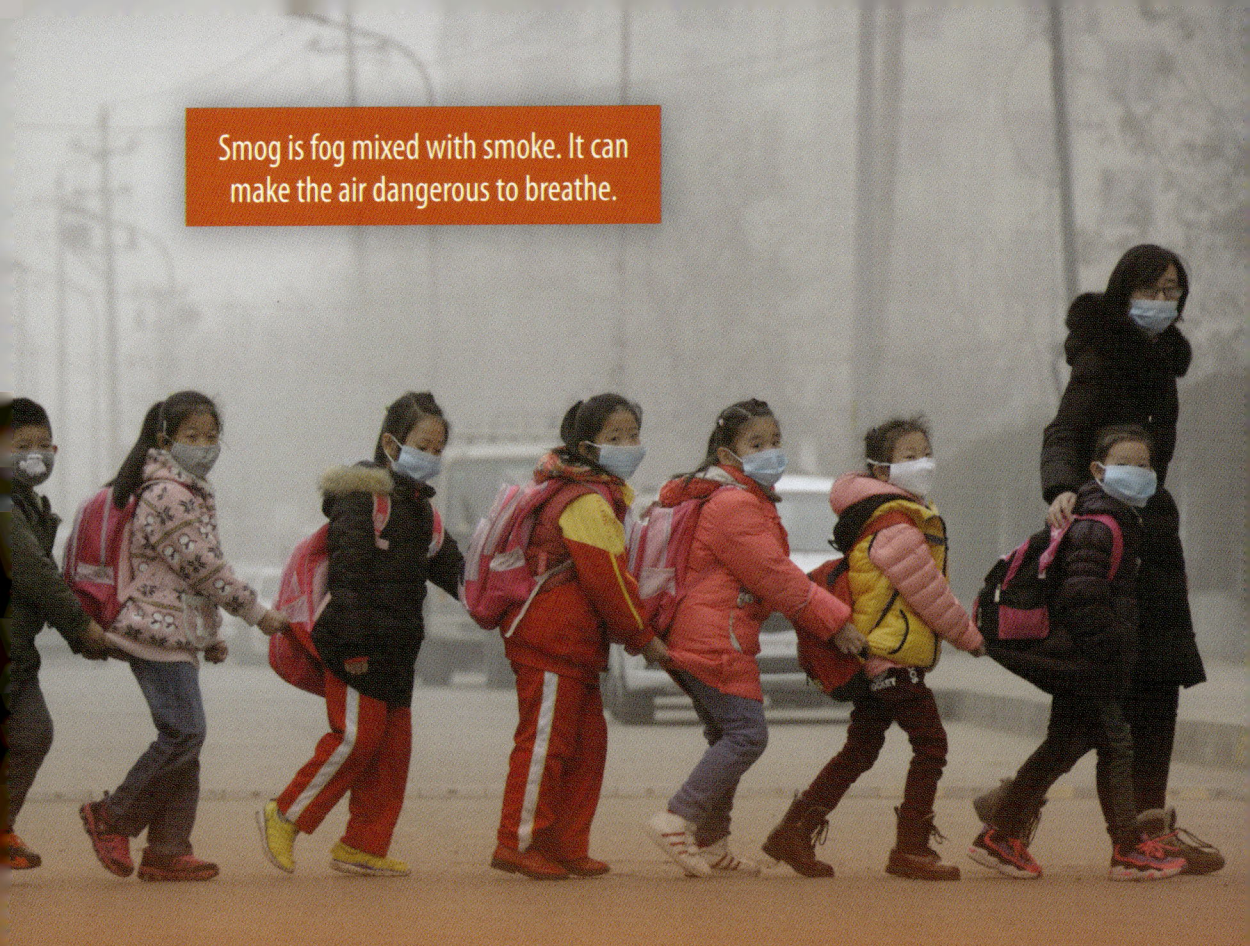

Smog is fog mixed with smoke. It can make the air dangerous to breathe.

There are two main kinds of pollution: ambient air pollution, which happens outdoors, and household air pollution. Cars, trucks, industries, and other things create ambient air pollution. Household air pollution mainly affects people in developing countries. Burning wood or coal at home produces smoke and pollution too.

CHAPTER TEN

THE IMPORTANCE OF NUTRITION

The World Health Organization (WHO) calls malnutrition one of the greatest challenges to world health. One form of this, called undernutrition, occurs when a person doesn't have enough food to live well. About 45 percent of deaths in children under five years old are related to undernutrition. About 462 million adults also suffer from undernutrition.

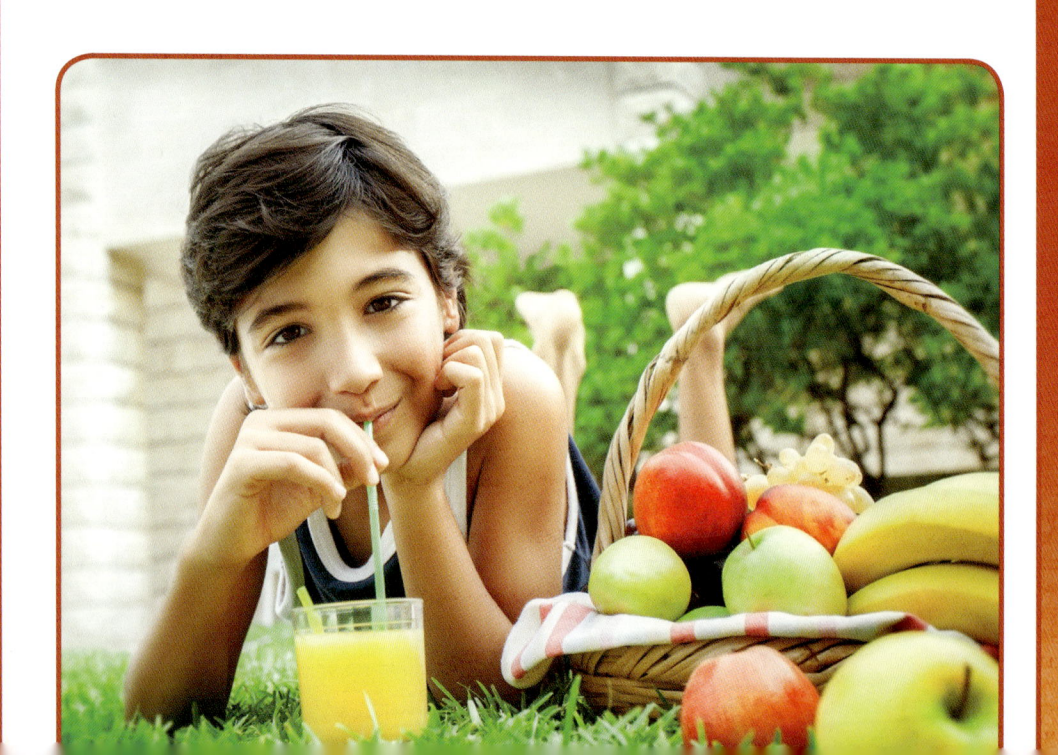

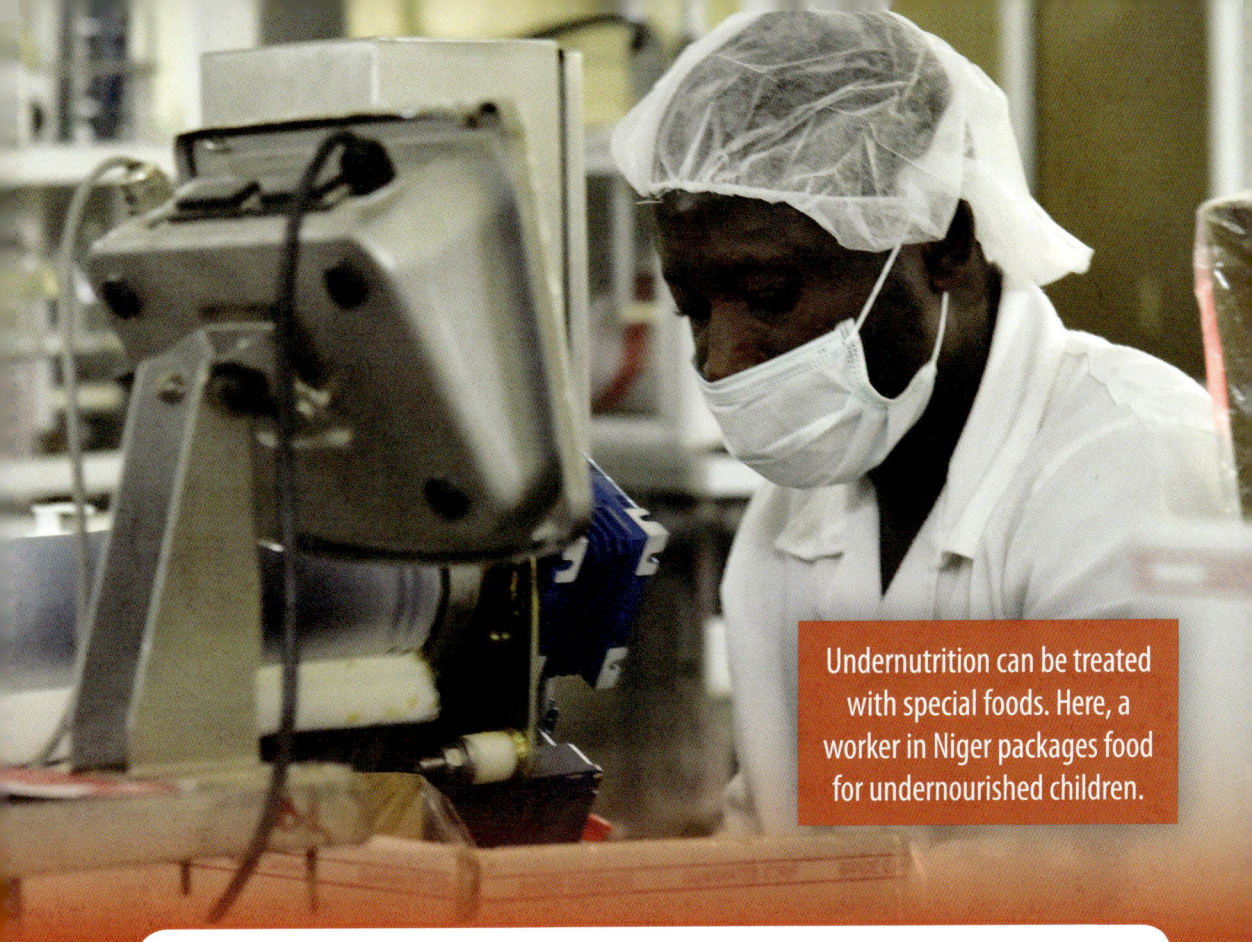

Undernutrition can be treated with special foods. Here, a worker in Niger packages food for undernourished children.

Another type of malnutrition happens when the body is missing certain vitamins or minerals, which are things that help keep people healthy. For example, some people don't have enough iron in their diets. Others might not have enough vitamin C.

Overweight people can suffer from malnutrition too. Even if someone gets enough food, it may not be high enough in nutrition to keep the person healthy.

CHAPTER ELEVEN

HEALTH OF MOTHER AND CHILD

Health care starts even before a child is born. It's important for **pregnant** women to receive healthy nutrition and care. They must also have a safe and healthy place and means to give birth. Both mothers and infants need to be treated by skilled providers before, during, and after birth.

Each year, thousands of mothers and infants die during or shortly after childbirth. Most of these deaths are preventable. Unfortunately, many people in developing countries can't reach trained health-care providers. They may live in areas without care facilities. In response, national and international organizations have pushed for better health care for women and babies. Most parts of the world have reduced the number of deaths connected with childbirth since 2000.

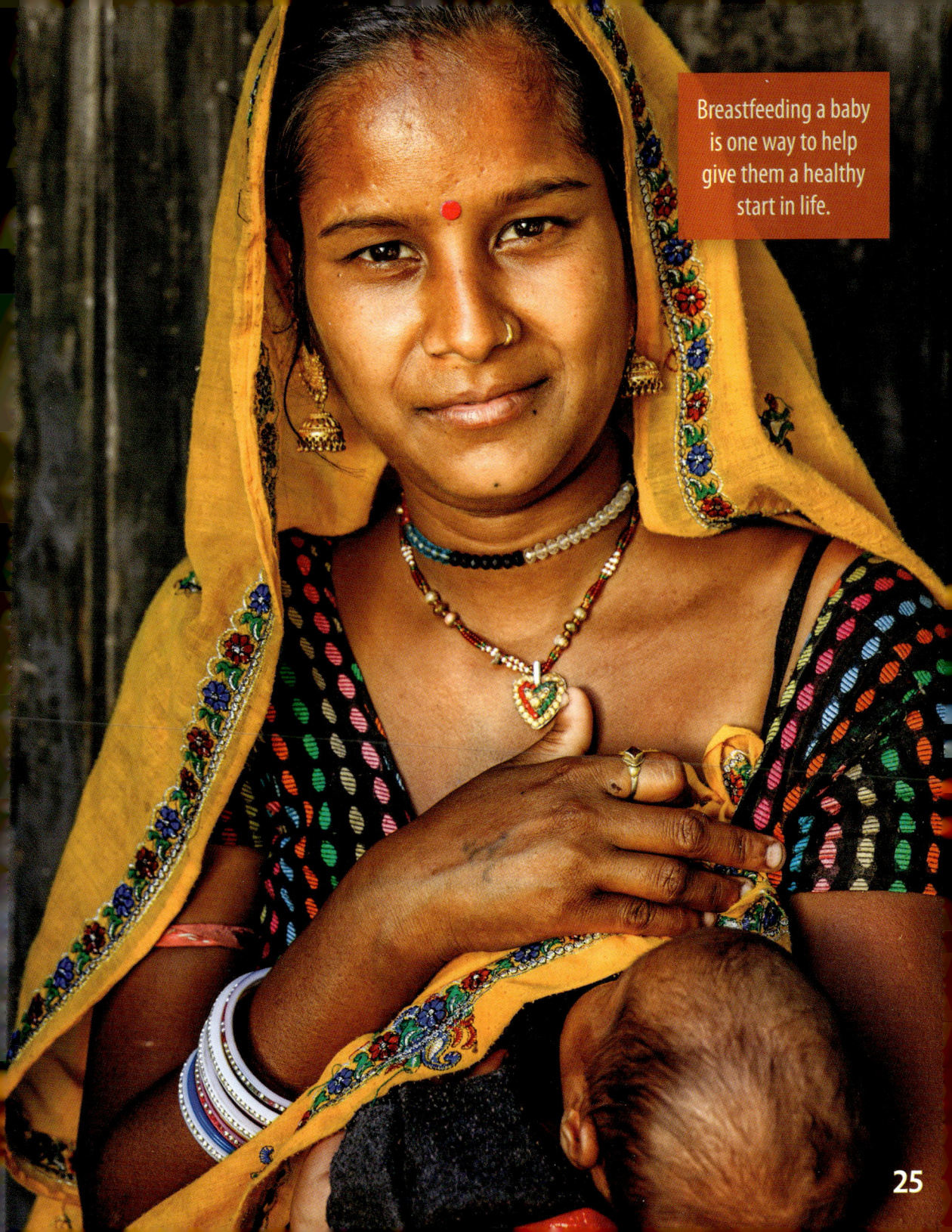

Breastfeeding a baby is one way to help give them a healthy start in life.

25

CHAPTER TWELVE

HEALTH CARE FOR ALL

It's hard to stay healthy when you can't see a doctor—and all health care costs money. Health-care coverage makes it possible for all people to get treatment when they need it. It's important that people of all income levels be able to have quality care.

Currently, about 1 billion people around the world don't have basic health-care coverage. In the United States, about 44 million people have no health insurance.

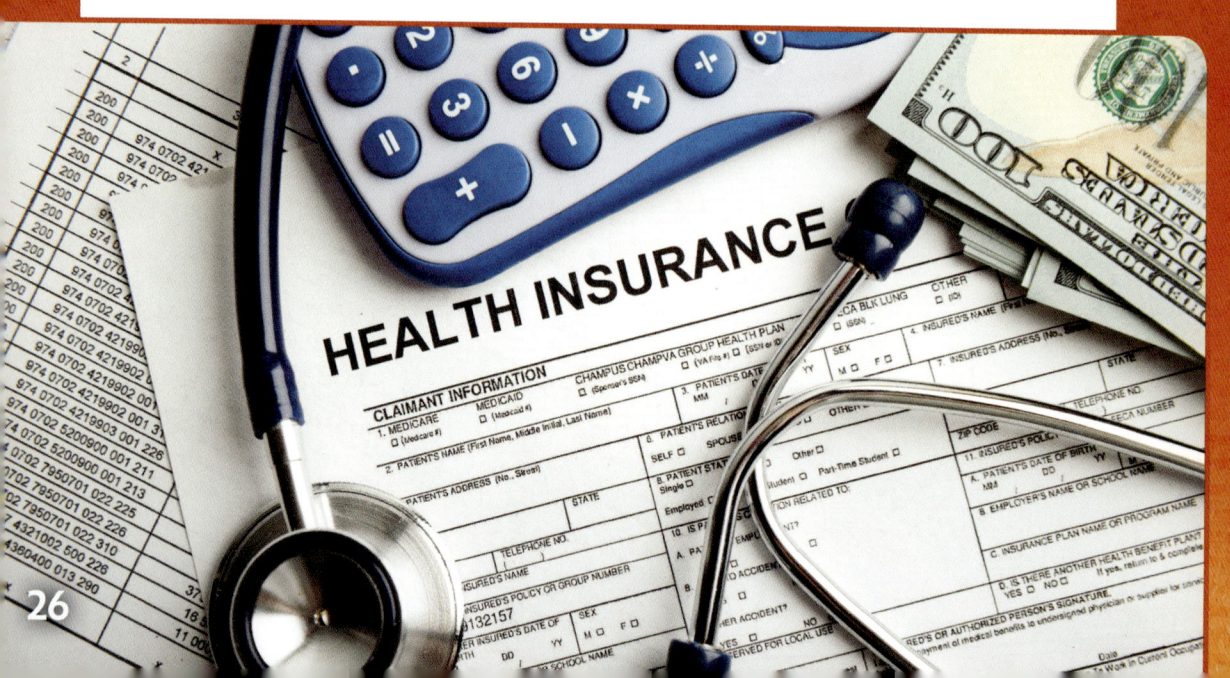

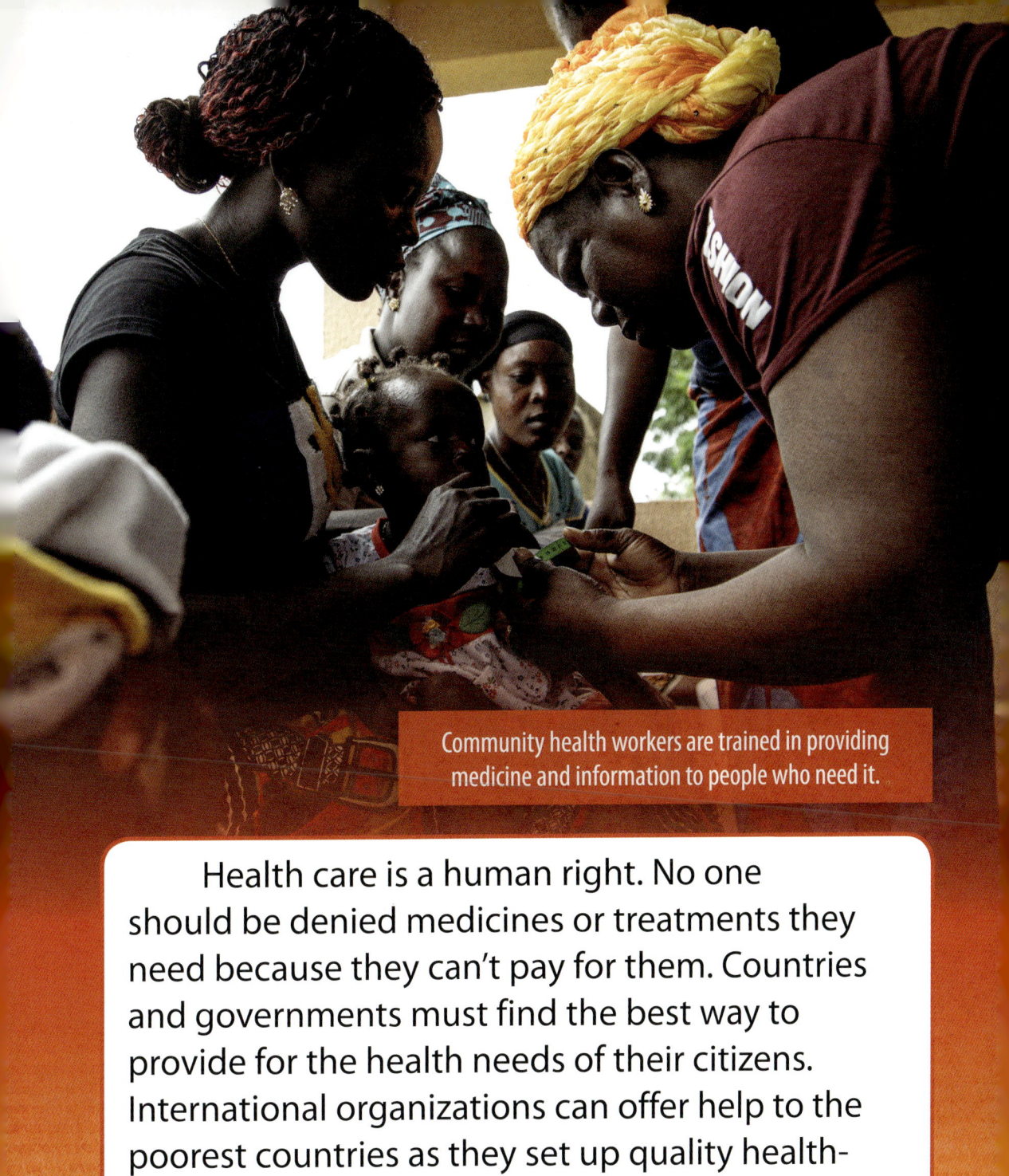

Community health workers are trained in providing medicine and information to people who need it.

Health care is a human right. No one should be denied medicines or treatments they need because they can't pay for them. Countries and governments must find the best way to provide for the health needs of their citizens. International organizations can offer help to the poorest countries as they set up quality health-care systems.

CHAPTER THIRTEEN

HEALTH CARE AND TECHNOLOGY

Technology has improved modern medicine. Doctors use new technologies in hospitals. Patients use technology to stay healthy. People have created over 160,000 health-related apps to track everyday behaviors, such as water intake and sleep. Using these mobile apps may make the users more likely to exercise. Taking these steps can help prevent diabetes and heart disease.

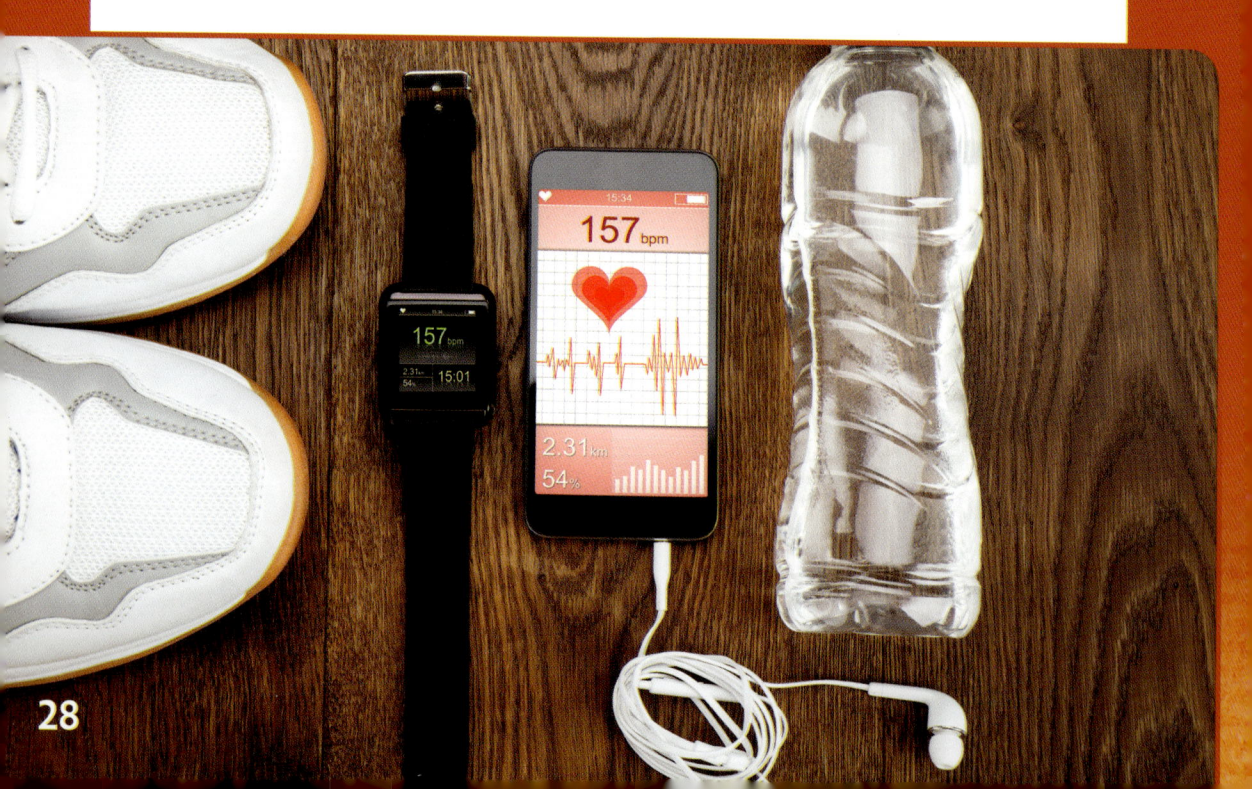

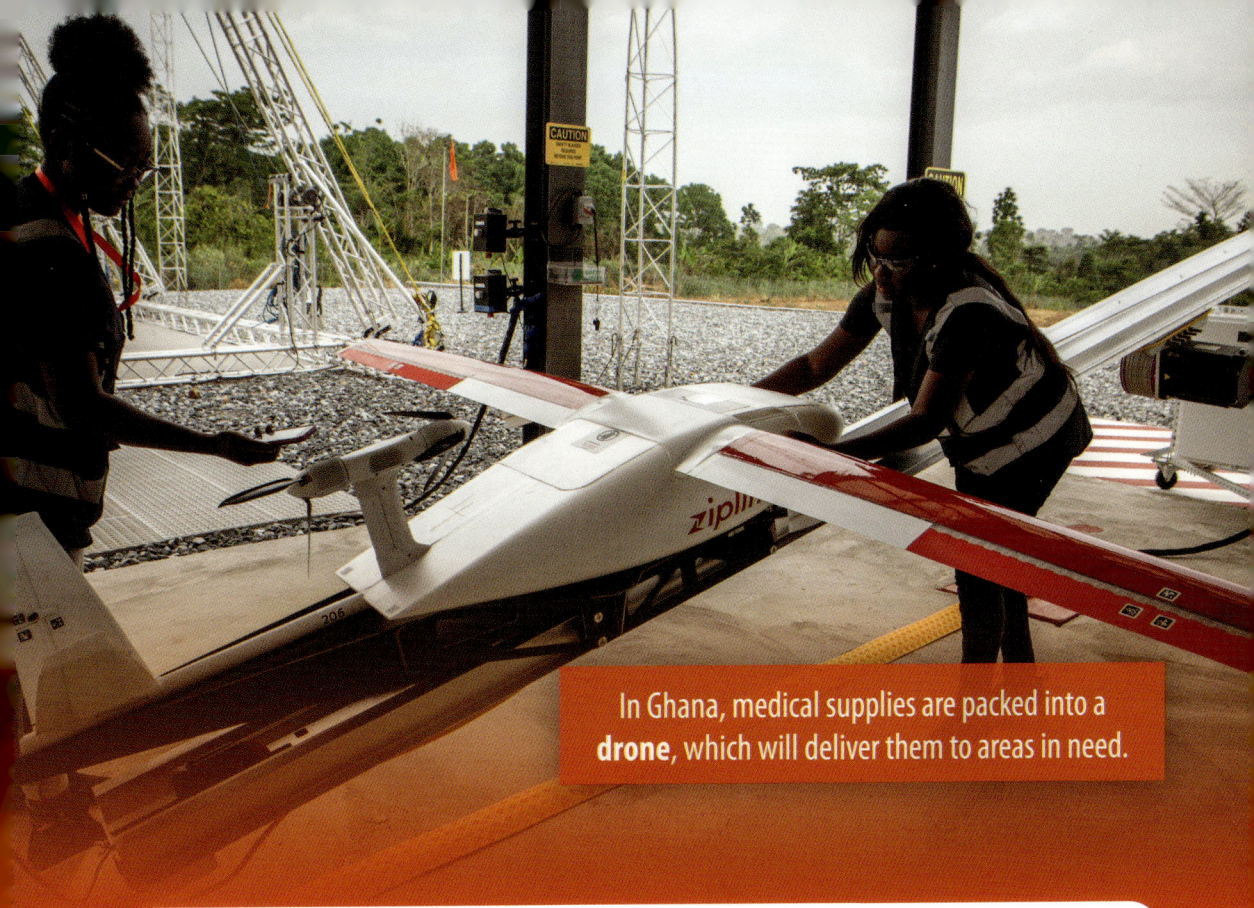

In Ghana, medical supplies are packed into a **drone**, which will deliver them to areas in need.

Mobile technologies such as video calling also help doctors and patients communicate. This can bring medical services to hard-to-reach areas. In Bangladesh, a program called Teledaktar provides virtual doctor appointments. Operators connect patients with volunteer doctors in other locations. Using video calling, the doctor can answer health questions. The doctor can also write **prescriptions** and send patients to specialists near them who can help.

CHAPTER FOURTEEN

TAKING ACTION

Improving physical health around the world is a large task. However, young people are doing a lot to help. Nujeen Mustafa was born with cerebral palsy, a condition that made her unable to walk. When she was 16, Mustafa fled from Syria to escape **conflict**. She journeyed 3,500 miles (5,632.7 km) to Germany. She traveled by bus, train, boat, and land. Mustafa made the whole trip in her wheelchair.

The trip convinced Mustafa that people needed to be aware of the needs of people with disabilities. Since then, Mustafa has addressed world leaders about planning for problems for people with disabilities. Mustafa's story shows that young people can help improve the world!

You can also make healthy choices for your body. Exercising and eating nutritious food can lead to better physical health in the future.

GLOSSARY

conflict (KAHN-flikt) A struggle between different forces.

drone (DROHN) A pilotless aircraft.

environment (ihn-VIY-ruhn-muht) The natural world around us.

genetics (juh-NEH-tiks) The genetic makeup of an organism.

insulin (IN-suh-luhn) A hormone in the body that helps process glucose, or sugar.

nutrient (NOO-tree-uhnt) Something taken in by a plant or animal that helps it grow and stay healthy.

pandemic (pan-DEH-mihk) An outbreak of a disease that affects a large amount of people all over the world.

paralysis (puh-RAA-luh-suhs) The state of being unable to move.

parasite (PEHR-uh-syt) A living thing that lives in, on, or with another living thing and often harms it.

plague (PLAYG) A disease that spreads from person to person quickly and kills many people.

pregnant (PREG-nuhnt) Having a baby developing inside the body.

prescription (prih-SKRIP-shuhn) A written message from a doctor that tells a patient to use a certain medicine or treatment.

technology (tek-NAH-luh-jee) A method that uses science to solve problems and the tools used to solve those problems.

INDEX

PRIMARY SOURCE LIST

Page 7
Bust of Hippocrates of Cos. Marble sculpture. Created circa 460 to 377 BC. Museo Archeologico Nazionale (Archaeological Museum). Naples, Italy.

Page 9
Microscope. Circa 1670. Created by Anton van Leeuwenhoek.

Page 11
Landing at Ellis Island. Photomechanical print. 1902. Library of Congress. Wikimedia Commons.

WEBSITES

Due to the changing nature of Internet links, PowerKids Press has developed an online list of websites related to the subject of this book. This site is updated regularly. Please use this link to access the list: www.powerkidslinks.com/SOOF/physical